YOUR HEALTH IS YOUR WEALTH

60 Inspirations for Fitness, Motivation and Resilience

Pam Sherman

Cover design by SoTold

Pam Sherman
Visit my website at www.theperfectbalance.guru

Printed in the United States of America

First Printing: January 2019
The Perfect Balance by Pam Sherman

ISBN: 9781793272775

Disclaimer:
This book and The Perfect Balance (theperfectbalance.guru) offer encouraging health, fitness and nutritional information and are designed for educational purposes only. You should not rely on this information as a substitute for, nor does it replace, professional medical advice, diagnosis, or treatment. If you have any concerns or questions about your health or starting an exercise regimen, always consult with a physician or other health care professional first.

This book is dedicated to the women who inspired me on my fitness journey. First, Cherie Lamb, my friend who clearly saw how much I loved fitness and told me about a course through Ohlone College. This was how to be an instructor. Next, Robin Kuratori, the instructor of that course. She taught me everything about formatting a class, from the music to how the class should be structured. Finally, Glenda Smith. She was my first boss who made me the instructor I became. I still hear her words today - learn your students' names. Thank them for coming. They can do anything in their day and they are choosing to come to your class. These fabulous women shaped me in my fitness career.

CONTENTS

INTRODUCTION

I've always loved moving my body. Once I became a group exercise instructor, I shared that love with my students. I always tried to make classes fun and challenging. My students left my class feeling accomplished, strong, and proud of their efforts.

Along the way (over the last 20 years) I would have contests in my classes - eat more veggies, drink more water, move more. I always tried to inspire them to put their health on their priority list and know they can feel great in their own skin.

When I was unable to teach after my accident, I still wanted to share my love of health and wellness. Starting my weekly emails, "The Perfect Balance Bulletin," was the perfect way to do this. This book is a compilation of those emails. I found inspiration all around me - from the guy who's checking me in to get my car fixed, to a person wanting to know the real deal on the latest diet.

I just want to share what I know to be true. Your health is your greatest wealth. There is nothing more important than taking care of yourself.

Read one entry each morning for 60 days - and repeat! We all benefit from daily reminders. I hope I inspire you to prioritize your health every single day!

BE POSITIVE

I want to talk about being positive today. Most of the clients I've worked with over the last 20 years have been women. They are absolutely awful to themselves. The negativity that comes out of their mouths is staggering.

"I need to lose weight," "I feel fat," "My arms/legs are jiggly" and so on. You may have said these things to yourself. It's so sad to hear.

Every single time this happens, I ask my client to say something positive about herself. Sometimes she can't even think of one thing. I could tell her at least 10 great things about her right then on the spot. I hate the fact that so many women have such awful self-worth.

Just for today – be positive. No negative self-talk. You *are* enough. You *are* awesome. You *are* amazing. Do not let one negative thought about yourself or your body take up one second in your head. Think of what your best friend would say about you – I'm certain she'd have more than one thing to say. In fact, she'd have a list of fabulous things about you.

Now, text a few of your friends something positive about them and make their day! Be positive about yourself – you are *amazing*!

GRATITUDE

In our instant gratification society, it is hard to be grateful sometimes. There is the FOMO (Fear Of Missing Out) when we look at what our friends are doing on Instagram or Facebook.

Life is not about FOMO, my friends. It's about your family and friends and health and wellness. We all have so much to be thankful for every single day.

I think we are all hard-wired to want more. A better job, more money, just more stuff. That's not really what makes us happy. It may for a moment, but certainly not long term.

Being healthy and being able to move our bodies feels awesome every single day. I see most of us take that for granted on a daily basis. It's not until we get an injury that we really are grateful for our healthy bodies. So get out and get moving today!

Having a great family and friends is paramount to happiness. Live people matter - not hundreds that like your picture on the internet. People that give you love and support and make you laugh till you cry are the ones that bring happiness. Even your pets bring you happiness - I know our pets bring my family tremendous joy.

How about a full set of teeth? I've got to throw that one out there! Can you bite into an apple today? If so be thankful. I am not joking -I am a long way off from being able to do that.

How about a job that you really love doing? Most of us take great pride in our work. A job well done brings us joy - this is something to be thankful for. If you don't have this - go out and find it.

Life is too short to think of what we don't have. Be thankful today for all you *do* have in your life.

Your health is your wealth!

PROGRESS, NOT PERFECTION

Not one of my clients will not be surprised to see this topic. I have said this to every single one of them over the years – we are *all* too hard on ourselves (myself included). This is true in so many aspects of our lives.

I see it too much with my clients regarding their food or exercise. Just about every single woman I have worked with beats herself up *way too much* about what she eats, as well as her exercise (or lack thereof).

I am here to tell you that I do not want you to be perfect. It is not attainable. It just makes you feel like crap when you are human and not perfect.

I would much rather see you be consistent and moderate rather than trying to reach food/workout goals that are just never going to happen.

Consistency is the key to lifelong health and wellness. Build habits that you can maintain daily all year long. This will make you feel like a rock star. Beating yourself up for what you didn't do just doesn't do you any good - it just stresses you out!

Easy things you can do to be consistent all year long:

1. Aim for 30 minutes of movement every day. This includes walking - it does not have to be an all-out kill yourself workout. But you absolutely can move your body for 30 minutes every single day. Not motivated? Check out YouTube for a million different workout videos.

2. Drink more water than you are right now. It's really hard in the winter or when it's rainy, but water is vital to our bodies - so drink up, buttercup!

3. Eat more vegetables every single day. One of my favorite health gurus I follow suggested 1 pound of raw veggies and half a pound of cooked veggies every day. Yikes! I just want you to think about having more than you are now, and include them in two out of your three meals a day.

Please don't strive for perfection ever. Just do better than you did yesterday, and be happy with that!

MASTER THE DAY

I saw a post on Instagram a few days ago that said:

You are not going to master the rest of your life in one day. Just relax. Master the day. Then just keep doing that every day.

It seems like everyone wants instant gratification. These are things I have heard people say over the years - mostly in jest, but with a hopeful word behind each one:

I have eaten great this week - why didn't I lose 5 lbs?
I started lifting weights, why don't my muscles show?
I finally am exercising a few times a week but don't see any results!

You get the picture. With our fast paced lives, it is understandable to expect immediate results for anything we undertake. I see this all the time with clients and friends in regards to food and fitness.

I want you to think about your health not just in the short term. Long term good health requires a lifelong commitment to eating well and moving your body.

How do you want to feel next month? Next year? In 10 years?

Put time and effort into your health today, and the next day, and the next. You will be rewarded for years to come. We are all a culmination of our choices in life. If you want to feel better - do something about it. It may be hard, but nothing worth having comes easy. You are worth it - make yourself and your health a priority every day.

THE BIG 5-0

Today I am the BIG 50! WOW!

I've read a few things over the last week that talked about our purpose. We are all put on this Earth to share our passion and to help others. It's the same message from various people that I follow, and it's hitting me over the head like a big hammer!

I truly believe I was put here on earth to share my love of fitness and a healthy lifestyle with all of you. I hope to influence many more as the years go by.

I have always loved to move my body and tortured my earliest friends (sorry Kelly and Cheryl) into running with me even though they didn't want to. Luckily, they've forgiven me and we've been friends our whole lives.

The big reason I wanted to write today is I honestly believe my passion saved my life. For those that don't know me well or my story, I was hit by a car while running a while ago. My brain is good, my bones are great, my ligaments and tendons back to normal and the only thing missing are 6 teeth. This was a result of me eating the windshield.

My sports guru told me I would have been far worse off if I hadn't been in such excellent shape when I got hit. That is a scary thought. Let's just say I could have been far worse off if I didn't take care of myself.

So this birthday has a far different meaning for me. I don't care at all about the number - it's just a number. I'm just thankful that I am here. Still a mom and a wife and a friend and a teacher.

This is one reason I'm so passionate about you taking care of yourself and your health every single day. Who gets hit by a car and doesn't break any bones? Can walk with very little pain, not need any pain meds to deal with any body ailments? Is back running 6 weeks later? *This* gal does!

Don't say you'll start tomorrow. Start today - eat some greens, drink loads of water, move your body! I have a ton of videos you can do at home from 5-10 minutes long on my YouTube channel.

Celebrate yourself and your health every single day!

THE TRUTH ABOUT WEIGHT LOSS

I know many people assume that I've never struggled with my own weight. They think that just because I'm a trainer, I've had it easy and can eat whatever I want and never gain a pound.

That's so far from the truth it's comical. I ate and drank a lot in college and was 25 lbs heavier in less than a year. Subs, pizza, beer, dorm food were on the menu. Even though I never stopped running, it didn't matter - I ate too many calories, therefore, I gained weight.

In fact, I was at my heaviest for most of my college days even though I ran one or two marathons a year. I was eating more calories than I was burning. I was famished after long runs and couldn't stop eating. This showed up on my body.

I was in such denial that I actually asked my friends if there was something wrong with me. Something felt weird on my back - it was back fat rolling up and down my body as I ran. I am not making this up! Bottom line, you can't outrun your fork!

One year for Spring Break I took Dexatrim 2 times a day and had a salad for dinner – and lost weight. Then I put it all back on during my vacation. I've tried Hydroxycut to lose weight, and exercising for weight loss. In short, I've tried it all. I've been so frustrated with my weight gain at times it's been horrible.

I'm exactly like many of you. For many years, I was desperate for that one thing that would help me lose weight. "Give me the magic bullet please so I can be done with this madness!"

About 4 years ago I had an injury that prevented me from running and in the same time frame my dad died. It was stress upon stress upon stress. It was no surprise that I put on weight. I was miserable in my own skin. Here I was a personal trainer who didn't know how to lose weight. I felt like a fraud. It was awful.

And then I discovered the magic bullet – the secret to weight loss. Count your calories. That's it. When I used Myfitnesspal on a regular basis, didn't exercise too much, got in enough protein and veggies, I lost weight. I got all the health/fitness magazines for years and never read this.

You have to be in a calorie deficit to lose weight. That's all there is to it. It's not glamorous or sexy. You also have to be consistent day in and day out.

I cringe now when I hear people talk about losing weight in a short time for vacation. I just heard a gal say, "I want to lose 10 lbs in 2 weeks because I'm going to the beach." Well guess what? That weight will come right back on when you eat and drink all you want because you are on vacation.

If you have weight to lose, it's because you've eaten too many calories. That's all there is to it. Yes, our metabolism slows down a bit as we get older, but that's no reason to put on weight. There was a gal at my current gym that said to me when I was in my early 40's, "Just wait till you're 50 Pam, you'll have a roll of fat right around your belly like I do." I just turned 50 and do not have a roll of fat around my belly.

If weight loss is your goal, start keeping track of what you eat. Then after a week, decrease your total intake by 10-15%. Start small so you will see success. Big quick losses never stick. Slow and steady wins the weight loss game.

I've been through it all. Please don't try anything that any store is selling you, or anything online. If any of that stuff worked, we'd all have perfect bodies. So please stay away from green tea promises, Slimfast, any kind of pills - any stuff on any shelf will *not* help you lose weight, ever. Been there done that. The only thing that will is creating a calorie deficit.

MEASURE YOUR SUCCESS

I train mostly women and see so many get wrapped up in the number on the scale. I know this has certainly happened to me as well. How silly to let a piece of metal control our moods for the day!

There are so many factors that go into the number on the scale - how hydrated you are, how much salt was in the previous day, hormones, where you are in your cycle, stress, lack of sleep - honestly the list goes on and on and on.

My thought for those interested in weight loss is to take measurements. We all have areas that carry extra weight - take out your tape measure and take 3 places on your body and measure those spots. For most gals - it's waist, hips and thighs. Then do it again the following week.

Or take out a piece of clothing you love that may be a bit snug and try it on once a week. For those who really want to see the changes happening - take pics in a bathing suit every few weeks - you will be amazed at the progress!

If you are eating well, moving your body, getting enough water and sleep, you will see changes. If you are not - then be honest with yourself about your food. It's a calorie deficit that creates weight loss - plain and simple. It's work to get the weight off, but certainly worth it to feel better in your own skin. One that you have to live in day in and day out.

If you really want to know how much you're eating, log your food for a week onto Myfitnesspal. Don't change anything, just eat like you normally do. Then, if you're not seeing progress on the scale or the measurements, decrease your calories by 10-15%. This will lead to weight loss. It's not super-fast but in my experience, those that lose it quickly put it back on even faster. Slow and steady wins the weight loss game.

There is one more thing I want you to do. Make a goal or two. It needs to be realistic. For example, I want to lose 1 - 2 inches off my waist in 6 weeks. I want to fit into my shorts again. I want to lose 5 lbs by June 15. You get the picture.

What's hard to measure is ... "I want to feel better." Or, "I want to be more fit." Those are way too general. I'd rather have you make short-term specific goals so you find success. As opposed to, "I want to drop 40 lbs by the end of the year" - YIKES! Let's think about 5 lbs at a time please.

If you want to lose weight, please don't put your head in the sand. Have a starting point. Take measurements, take pictures, try on some clothes you want to fit back into. Then make a time frame for a short goal. Once you hit that goal you can build upon that and keep going if you need to.

Life is too short to be uncomfortable in your own skin. You are the only one responsible for what goes in the pie hole. If you want to see changes, make it happen.

TALK YOURSELF INTO IT

I want to talk about setting up daily healthy habits. I hear people often say, "I should go to the gym." "I should eat better." "I should drink less." "I should drink more water." The list goes on and on.

The only person holding you back from doing these things is ... you! We all have busy lives with long to do lists. Unfortunately, it's just the way life is these days.

Here's the key to setting up better habits - don't try to change too many things at once. I often tell my clients to change or add in one thing at a time. That is doable.

Trying to drink more water, eat more veggies, and get to the gym 4 times – all of these changes in one week - just shouts "unrealistic" and sets a person up for failure.

I hate taking things away from people. I would rather have them add good habits to their day. Pick one thing you really want to improve on - just one. Put that on the top of your to-do list for a week and you'll be amazed at your progress. Once you are successful, move on to the next good habit you want to tackle.

Need to drink more water? Set your alarm on your phone for every 2 hours during the day and finish your water bottle before the next alarm rings. Easy to implement.

Need to eat more veggies? Make a smoothie with a few handfuls of spinach (with a piece of fruit and some protein powder, water or almond milk) and have a big salad for lunch or dinner and BAM— you've just had 5+servings of veggies!

Need to move your body more? Get a pedometer - it doesn't have to be fancy. In fact, I got mine at Target for $16 and it clips onto my pants. See how much you move for a few days, then try to move more. Or do some of my videos in the comfort of your own home. YouTube also has thousands of videos to choose from as well!

We are only given one body to go through life with. It's our job, the most important job to take care of it every single day. If you are a parent, your kids need to see you doing this so they know how to take care of their own bodies as well!

Don't talk yourself out of taking care of yourself and your health. You are worth it - every single time. I promise, you will never regret a workout, drinking more water, or eating more veggies.

PITBULL

I'm not talking about the dog, but the singer and his song, *Time of My Life*. There are a few lines that so resonate with me.

This is for anybody going through tough times. Believe me, been there, done that. But everyday above ground is a *great* day - remember that.

We all go through tough times. People get sick and die. Accidents happen. Divorce from loved ones happens. Bad bosses, bad friends, bad family members, bad jobs, etc. It is just a part of life.

But how we deal with the bad times truly makes a difference in our everyday life. We can either be a victim of our circumstance – "woe is me, it's so terrible that X happened." Or – "shit happens," put a smile on your face, and get through it the best you can.

I'm not saying not to grieve a loss. But rather, stay positive and move forward. Life is so, so much better when you are not Debbie Darkcloud. My positive outlook since my accident is something many people comment on - weekly in fact. I'm a happy person for the most part and I truly believe life is better when you have an upbeat attitude.

At the end of the day - *every* day above ground is a *great* day. Believe me, my mantra since my accident is *better than dead.* I'm not joking, because I could have been killed.

We all have a choice every single day. How we face each day is up to you. Go out and make your own movie - be the star and the director and make it a killer day.

Now go out and make it an *amazing* day - because you *can!*

FAT LOSS

Fat loss ... does not happen in the gym. It happens the other 23 hours you are out of the gym.

You can't out-exercise a bad diet. What you can do is make small changes one day, one week at a time to see changes in your body.

I've seen too many people over the years spend too many hours in the gym and expect miraculous changes. To lose fat, you do not need a lot of time spent sweating. You need to create a calorie deficit.

If you exercise a lot, you get really hungry. Which leads to overeating. Which does not lead to fat loss.

Losing weight can be so overwhelming. So many different plans on the internet and quick fixes on the shelves (all of which are total crap - please don't buy any of it). What can a person do?

1. Don't try any quick fixes.
2. Make yourself and your health a priority every day.
3. Add one new habit a week. I never take away things from my clients but add good things in first.

- Week 1 - Drink more water.
- Week 2 - Eat more veggies.
- Week 3 - Move your body for 30 mins 3 times a week.
- Week 4 - Know that you are human. Do not aim for perfection. We all fall down. It's how you get back up and move on that counts.
- Week 5 - Enlist in the help of loved ones. Having a good support system is huge when trying to lose weight. Better yet, get a weight loss buddy and be accountable and challenge each other.

The national average for losing weight and keeping it off is 5%. 95% of people gain their weight back. That's not a great percentage.

Here's the thing - losing weight and adopting a different, healthier lifestyle is a lifelong commitment. 95% of people change their habits during the weight loss phase, then go back to their old way of life. No surprise the weight comes back on. This is a fork to mouth problem.

If you are not happy in your own skin, start with small steps. Be successful, then add on. You can change your habits for the better. You are the only one who can do it. You are worth it!

RESOLUTIONS

As I was out running today, I was wondering how many of you read last week's email and set up some short term goals?

I did! I needed to drink more water and run more. I had a plan and made it work. I printed out a calendar and wrote down if I ran and if I got in enough water. It felt really good make a plan and succeed. So far so good!

Today I thought about New Year's Resolutions. Such a big deal is made in January about changing our lives for the better. Getting into new habits and making them stick. At my gym, we always know the first two weeks in January are packed with newbies.

Then what happens? Reality, life, and to be honest – most people do not carry any resolutions much past the second week in January. The best intentions are forgotten. The gym clears out to the regulars by the third week in January – every single year.

Did you make a New Year's Resolution? Do you even remember what it was?

So, instead of making and breaking a New Year's Resolution. I want you to think of an end of the year Resolution. There's 7 months until the end of the year.

How do you want to change your health for the better?

Make a short list of things you'd like to incorporate into your life now so that by the end of the month, you'll feel really amazing about yourself and your health.

These do not have to be *huge* goals. Small ones work. I see far too many people struggle with their health and their weight on a daily basis. If you put down your goals now, and make an action plan, you can feel (both mentally and physically) a million times better. Get a clear idea of what you want for yourself and *go for it!*

We only get one body to go through life. How do you feel when you wake up? When you get dressed? When you go out shopping? When you exercise? When you look at yourself in the mirror?

If any one of these answers are less than pretty good, get on it and make some end of year's resolutions. I want you to love how you feel every single day. I want you to wake up without aches and pains. To fit into your clothes. To feel great when you move your body. To be your best self possible.

I had a different kind of resolution this year. My New Year's Resolution was to see my friends more often. That was it. After an event like my accident, I wanted to be around the people I loved most, more often. And I'm happy to say that is one resolution that I've kept!

Now it's your turn. Make a list of a few things you'd really like to accomplish. Make an action plan. List the things you need to do to be successful. How GREAT would it be to finish off the year working towards yourself and your health? I think it'd be pretty awesome.

EMOTIONAL EATING

What do you do when you are happy, sad, lonely, frustrated, upset, ecstatic? *Eat!*

We have become a nation of eating for every occasion. Think about it - there's never a reason not to eat these days and it shows. 70% of Americans are overweight or obese. 70%!

I get it, I've done it myself - heck who hasn't?

If you are looking to control your eating and lose some extra pounds, emotional eating has got to go. Let's just also say- no one is sitting down with a bag of apples when they are sad. It's chips/cookies/candy - all the stuff that makes us feel good for a minute. But also makes you go back for more and more and more.

I think that we are avoiding our feelings. I'm convinced that most if not all people that emotionally eat/overeat on a regular basis have other issues. I'm not talking about 20-30 lbs overweight. Obesity comes from many other issues such as depression.

We all like to eat, even love to eat. However, obesity comes from our emotional needs. It's easier to stuff our feelings down with food than deal with the reality of what is really bothering us.

Next time you want to eat yourself silly, ask yourself how you are feeling. I know for me, fatigue is my number one reason I overeat. I've been known to polish off far too many calories because I'm exhausted.

Does it make me less tired? No, of course not! Now I consciously ask myself - am I really hungry or tired? This just happened recently. I was starving! I had an awful night of sleep the night before. I knew I was really tired and not starving, so I took a nap. When I woke up I was not hungry.

What are you feeling? Bored? Go read a book. Need comfort? Call a friend or get some fuzz therapy. Angry - get outside and get moving. Lonely? Go out and be around other people. You get the picture.

We all have shit to deal with. Food will never ever resolve any emotional issues we have. Figure out what you need and get help if need be. Talking to a friend/loved one will always give you more comfort than a bag of chips or a box of cookies.

It's ok to feel your feelings. Cry, laugh, stomp around, swear, jump for joy - you get it. Feelings are meant to be felt, not eaten.

Make yourself and your health a priority every single day.

YODA

One of my son's favorite quotes is from the great Yoda– Do or Do Not – there is no *try*!

I was thinking about this recently as so many people try to make a shift in their lives.

Here's a few examples: I'm going to try to exercise more, I'm going to try to drink more water, I'm going to try to eat better, I'm going to try to log my food. You get the picture. Do or do not – there is no try.

I often think people try for too much at one time. My recent posts about goals come to mind. Pick 1-2 small goals that are attainable and make them happen. Trying to overhaul too much will just lead to failure.

You either do something or you don't.

Want to drink more water? Have a daily goal and track it. Want to add more veggies – plan out your meals every day and include veggies. Want to exercise more? Plan your day and figure out the best time for you to move your body.

It's important that you value yourself and your health. You are worth the effort. Once you know that, you absolutely are going to make the change (whatever that may be). There will be no try! You *will* do it!

LIMITS

We are all capable of so much more than we even know. Every single one of us. We put limits on ourselves all the time. I constantly hear people say ... I could never-run a marathon, get up early, exercise, lose weight, drink less alcohol, drink more water. Literally, the list goes on and on.

Why not? The only limit is you.

No one is holding you back from anything in life but yourself. Want to learn a new language? Learn an instrument? Everything is available to us through the internet.

Want to feel good in your body once and for all? Make small changes daily that leads to long term success.

Nothing is out of your reach. We all have busy lives. Every single one of us. But there is time for the things we want to get done every single day.

I *love* when someone tells me they don't have time to exercise or eat right. I bust every excuse every single time. I will quote the great Jimmy Ryan (my high school cross-country coach) again and again- "Excuses are like assholes. Everyone has one and they all stink."

So what do you want to accomplish? Make a 3 month plan on how you will tackle this and then put it into place. The worst words ever are *I can't*. You pretty much *can* do anything you put your mind to.

Reach for the stars!

CHANGE

Change is hard. Sometimes scary. Most don't like it. But it happens all the timen- sometimes daily.

Big changes are tough to handle that is for sure. Little changes seem easy by comparison.

We all deal with change differently. Some roll with it, some fight it. But it comes no matter what.

It brings up a quote from the movie Cousins - this movie is from 1989 - but I've always remembered this particular line:

"You've only got one life to live. You can either make it chicken shit, or chicken salad."

You only have one life to live! Are you satisfied with yourself and your health? If not, do something about it today. You are the *only* one who has 100% control of this. I want you to fight for your own health on a daily basis. Move your body, drink more water, eat lots of veggies, and don't settle for anything less than the best!

AFTER A FALL

Life has its ups and downs. One day can be awesome and the next day awful. That's just the way it goes.

The good times are easy and fun. Who doesn't love to have things go your way? Celebrate your success? Feel amazing about something you've accomplished?

Then the bad times come and shit hits the fan. Something awful happens. This is a part of life and none of us are exempt unfortunately. We will all fall down and have to deal with really harsh situations.

It's easy to have a pity party and get depressed about the situation. I promise you it will be better for your mental health to look at the bright side and be as strong as possible.

If you don't, you'll just look like a toddler having a temper tantrum! It's not easy, it's not fun, but you will come out stronger on the other side if you hold your head up high and do everything you can to move forward with a positive attitude.

We all fall down; it's how we pick ourselves back up that shows our true character. Be strong, ask for help, and know it will pass eventually.

TIME

It's back to school time for kids. Where does the time go?

Just a few years ago I was sending my boy to kindergarten and yesterday I dropped him off for his second year in college.

Time - you can't stop it, you can't make it go faster or slower, you can only make the best of it.

What are you doing to make the best use of your time for your health?

I hear people all the time and have for years and years tell me, it takes too much time to eat right, exercise - fill in the blank with anything related to living a healthier life.

I'm calling bullshit on that. We all make time for things we want to do. I'm so passionate about this because I know if you put the time and effort into yourself, you will feel better today, tomorrow and even 10 years from now.

If you don't - you will struggle. It'll be hard to get out of bed, you will have low energy, you will have aches and pains you wouldn't have if you put the time into yourself and your health.

The choice is yours. Time will pass regardless. I vote for making your health your top priority every single day. You are worth it. I believe it's the single most important thing you can do for your present and your future.

PUT YOUR HEALTH FIRST

Over the 20 years of training and teaching, I've heard it all. Every excuse in the book. Probably the most common one is "I can't." As in *I can't* find the time to workout, *I can't* figure out how to eat better, *I can't* because of the kids/husband - and the list goes on and on.

I'm here to tell you that you *can*. I find that people fail because they try to make too many changes at one time. They try to start a new exercise regime and totally new diet plan, and expect perfection that first week. That will lead to disaster every single time.

Here's how you find success. Try one small change this week. Seriously. If you don't drink a lot of water, drink a few more glasses a day. If you do not move your body, get out and walk 15 mins a day. If you don't get enough fruit/veggies, eat one apple every day.

Incorporate whatever you need to every single day. Seems small right? But you will feel awesome and accomplished if you make this small change. By doing this, you are building up a good habit, one habit at a time. This will lead to the next small change. Small steps = success.

We all have habits we can improve on – yep – every single one of us. I promise that making small changes will lead to long term success. One thing at a time and know that nothing is impossible!

The quote a journey of 1,000 miles begins with a single step is a perfect reference here. A healthy lifestyle begins with one habit at a time. I know you can do this!

YOU NEVER KNOW

You never know what you can do until you try. We have all probably heard this from our parents at some point or another. If you are a parent, you have probably said this to your child. It is so true.

I was running with a friend last week and we were talking about limits. We were talking about little kids who climbed a tree at her school. Some kids were daredevils and climbed really high. Some were not and only climbed up a bit. Some were not even going to try.

This can apply to us all. There will always be new situations in our lives. How will you act is up to you!

Will you charge ahead and go for the top branch?

Will you be scared and get to the bottom branch and think that's enough. Or turn away from it all and think, I can't do that.

The only limit is the one we place on ourselves. I really hate the word *can't*. It's self-imposed failure. Every time I hear that, it's honestly just another excuse. You *can* do anything you want.

What if the next time a challenge came your way and instead of being scared or talking yourself out of it, you thought – hell yes, I'll give it a go?

I would rather see you try and fail than not try at all. Life is more fun when you put yourself out there and try something new. Take a risk – you never know what could happen unless you try.

SILVER LINING

Today for the first time since my accident, I ran to the place where I got hit. For those that don't know this, I was hit by a car while running not too long ago. I was just in the wrong place at the wrong time. Simple as that. Bad things happen in life and this was one of them.

I have driven by this spot several times, but not been up for actually running there. To say it was emotional is an understatement. I had to stop and let myself give in to my emotion. It's the first time I have let myself really absorb what happened to me.

I know that sounds odd, but I'm an inherently optimistic person. I honestly could have been killed. I'm so thankful I'm not dead, not in a wheelchair, and/or not brain damaged. What could have been life threatening was just life changing.

Life is funny - you get ups and downs. You always hear, "there's a silver lining behind every dark cloud." Kind of corny, but in this case true. I've not ever given one thought to *why me?* What's the point? Bad stuff happens to everyone.

In this case, I've started something I've wanted to do for a long time. Reach more people. Since I was unable to teach classes after my accident - I thought - what a perfect time to start a website! I thought about making videos 15 years ago - in the VHS time. But back then, had no clue how I could even make that happen.

My friend had a fantastic woman who helped with her website and BAM! The Perfect Balance was born!

Since then I've authored a few books, and launched a new online coaching program, "Sexy in 60 Days." Seriously - I never would have done any of this if I hadn't left my house exactly when I did last December.

I think it's easy to get caught up in the bad. Have a pity party. Be a victim. But we all have a choice. Stew in misery or move on to better things. I vote for moving on to better things. Life is so much better with a positive outlook!

KINDNESS

It has been heartwarming to see the kindness of others on the news. Anywhere there's been a natural disaster, where people are losing everything, they are still helping others. The stories come in non-stop.

It doesn't matter what political party you are, what socioeconomic group you are in, what color you are, people are just helping people. Sometimes it takes the worst to bring out the best.

It does feel good to be kind, to do acts of service, just to help out. I always try to help older people with their carts, new moms at a door, or just when I see someone needs it. It is never a big deal to me but it is always appreciated.

So why is it so easy to be kind to others, and not ourselves? I mostly work with women. As a whole, we are unkind to ourselves daily. The things I hear women say about themselves are harsh and very critical. The negative that comes out of their mouths, far outweighs the positive.

Those of you who know me, know my standard response when I hear an unkind remark. OK - now say something nice about yourself. Sometimes people take a long time to think of one thing.

This is awful. We should be able to think of many positive things right away!

Make a list right now of 5 positive things about yourself. Put it on a sticky note and look at it daily. So the next time you say something awful (unfortunately this is not very often for many), think of your list.

You are awesome, you are fabulous, you are kind, you are funny ... you are amazing!

I have a friend I've known for 45 years. Her name is Kelly. IT's her birthday is today. She is one of the kindest people I know. A special birthday shout out to her on a day most people think about 9/11 - another tragic event that brought out the best in people trying to recover from tragedy. If more people were as kind as Kelly, this world would be a much better place.

Make yourself and your health a priority every single day!

FINISH WHAT YOU STARTED

Last night I was thinking about the run that I didn't finish. (Also known as a "DNF" for my running friends.)

The day I got hit, I was out for a 6.5 mile run. I've not run that far since then. But thought it was time. Time for closure and finish that damn run.

As I set out this morning to do just that, it occurred to me it was exactly 9 months ago. Only recently have I been putting in enough miles to finish this run. It was a perfect morning. Cool with no breeze. I finished what I started.

More often than not, I see people *not* finish what they have started. This is in regards to their health/fitness goals. Drink more water, exercise more, log their food, eat more veggies, be accountable – you get the picture. It's always easy to start, exciting even, but really hard to finish.

Why is that? Why are we so eager to set goals and rarely meet them?

I've seen both my kids make goals and reach them which is awesome. My son had put on some weight his freshman year in college. He didn't like the way he felt in his own skin and dropped it. I am super proud of him. I put on 30 lbs my first year at OSU and it took me years to take off. He did it in just a few months.

My daughter follows lots of soccer players on Instagram. One of them, Emily Boyd (who is a keeper at Cal) talks a lot about healthy eating. Emily recently said she's giving up processed carbs for a month. Think bread, tortillas, cookies, chips etc. My girl is a great eater but wanted to challenge herself to do the same thing. She's doing it because she really wants it. Just like my son did. I am super proud of them both.

I think that's really the key to any goal you set for yourself. You really have to want it, really want it and be willing to make the sacrifices along the way to get there. Reaching goals is never an easy process that is for sure.

I challenge you right now to make a goal. Short term. Something you have wanted to do for a long time now but just have not made happen. Make it a small goal please. Even just something for 14 days. But, you really can do anything you put your mind to for 14 days.

"By the end of 14 day, I want to ..." you fill in the blank. Now think about the steps needed to make it happen. Now do it.

And if you really do make it happen, I'd LOVE to know about it. I always love success stories and see people accomplish things they want to. Especially in regards to their health.

THE FINISH LINE

We all work hard for things we do in life. Tests in school, jobs, races/sporting events, raising kids, working out - the list is endless. As well as dieting.

I have seen many people lose weight over the years on a diet. They are all successful. If you follow a plan, any plan it will 100% work for you. Atkins works, Weight Watchers works, low fat works, Nutri-system works, the Whole 30 works.

But these are all short term. I'd say 95% of the people (if not more) have regained all the weight they lost (sometimes more) on the diet when they got to the finish line - their goal weight.

You see, with health and fitness there is NO finish line. This is something you need to do for the rest of your life. We are meant to move, not be sedentary. So get up and get moving every single day. We are made up of between 50-65% water so drink water every day. We are supposed to eat foods grown from the ground. Much more than foods from a package. Try to eat more fresh food every day.

Your health truly is your wealth. There are so many chronic diseases that are caused from our diet - obesity, diabetes, cardiovascular disease, some forms of cancer, osteoporosis and so many more. We can truly change the last part of our lives with how we treat our bodies today and tomorrow and the day after that and the year after that.

There is *no* finish line in the health game of life. Take care of yourself and your health every single day.

EVERY CHOICE WE MAKE

I am passionate about healthy eating and exercise. Those of you that know me can vouch for this. Those of you that don't - well let's just say it's spot on!

Both my father and my father in law died of food related diseases. This makes it really important for me to spread the word of eating well for life long health. My dad died from complications of Alzheimer's - which is being called Type 3 Diabetes now. My father-in-law died from issues related to obesity.

None of us are getting out of this world alive, but I'm certain we could have had more years with these amazing men, had they made better food choices in the years prior to their deaths.

I came across a quote the other day that summed up exactly how I feel, and I'll leave you with it today.

"Every meal is s short-term investment in how you feel and perform, a mid-term investment in how you look, and a long-term investment in your freedom from disease." - Alan Aragon.

THE KETO DIET

There's always a popular diet going around. In the 70's - Atkins, 80's and 90's - low fat, high carb and more recently the Paleo diet as well as the High Protein diet. I'm seeing and hearing a ton of questions about the Keto diet.

If you've not heard of it, the Keto diet is very high fat. 75-80% of your food comes from fat, moderate protein and super low carbohydrate. This diet is really great for Parkinson's disease as well as epileptics.

It's been all over social media lately and I've had no less than 5 people in the last week ask me about it. I am not a doctor or nutritionist but I want to tell you my thoughts on this diet.

It's ridiculous. It's not something you can do for the rest of your life. On the keto diet you cannot have any pizza, birthday cake, bread, potatoes, rice, most fruit or much fun - lol. It's not going to help you lose weight long term if that is what you are looking to do.

Are you really not going to have a piece of cake or cookie ever again? Say no to a banana because it has too many carbs?

No one got fat eating bananas!

Come on my friends – you are better than this! No diet works for the rest of your life. Diets *do* work in the short term Life – long health and a maintaining a healthy weight is what we are talking about here. To do that, eat real food – yep even bananas and apples and berries and watermelon, peaches, plums, pears, and even carrots!

I am convinced there is no food that is grown from the ground that you should avoid ever. There was no obesity epidemic in the early to mid-1900's. They were only eating real food. No packaged crap – there was none!

My goal here is to steer you away from diets and learn to eat real food. Eating should be enjoyable and satiating. Healthy eating and a moderate weight can do wonders for your health now and for the rest of your life!

PERSPECTIVE

I was recently at a friend's house and heard a crazy story about a woman at a gymnastics meet. She made a huge scene because her daughter (who placed 3rd in an event) got her medal, but it was not announced over the loudspeaker. This mom proceeded to say it was the worst day of her (10 year old) daughter's life and ranted on and on and on. To the point, she actually embarrassed her daughter.

This struck me as ridiculous. I can understand her being disappointed but making scene about something like that just seem trivial compared to what is happening all around us. I live in Northern California about 2 hours away from the horrible fires that have taken far too many lives and homes. In fact, 25 girls were not at this meet because they lost their homes.

Things like this happen all the time. People make mountains out of molehills. I actually felt sorry for the mom. What about the phrase - don't sweat the small stuff. People have lost so much - and she's worried about an announcement. Really?

Look at the bigger picture always. Think of the things you are thankful for. That's today message. Be thankful you have a home, you are alive, you have your health and you have your family. The other stuff just doesn't matter.

THEME SONG

Whenever I hear a song from the 80's, I instantly think about where I was when that song came out. So many fun high school and college memories float around The Cure, Depeche Mode, Book of Love, Journey, The Outfield and the list goes on and on.

I'm guilty of not always knowing the meaning behind most songs. Music just makes me happy. Many times I'll sing along to the radio and not really think about the story behind the song.

Last week when I heard Survivor by Destiny's Child, I thought – damn that should be my theme song! I have survived a lot. Tumultuous home life as a kid, dad living by me in his last years – declining and fighting Alzheimer's/Dementia, getting hit by a car last year. I *am* a survivor!

What's your theme song? What really resonates with you when you hear it? I'd love to know.

If you are ever *not* in the mood to workout/move your body, just put on your favorite upbeat song and you will be motivated to get out the door and get moving!

HEROES

Since tomorrow is Halloween and lots of kids will dress up in superhero costumes, I wanted to talk a bit about heroes.

I just saw a kid last night at my daughter's soccer practice in the full Spider-Man muscle costume. My son had one just like it many years ago, and wore it until it had holes in it!

If you ask a kid who their hero is, it's easy to get an answer. Wonder Woman, Spider-Man, Batman - the list is endless. You may even get a mom or dad answer as well.

I think it's much harder as an adult to have a hero. We grow up and see our folks as fallible. They are not perfect and actually make mistakes. It is also harder because our expectations are so much higher than when we were kids.

What if for one day - you made yourself your own hero. Make a list of everything you want to be - and work towards that list for one day. If you feel amazing, keep it going.

What could that list contain?

- Strength - mental and physical

- Superpower - we *all* have them- you just have to look for yours (my family says mine is being able to sleep on planes - LOL)
- To be Unstoppable - So many people are their own worst critics and sabotage their own efforts. Get out of your own way and shoot for the stars!
- To be the Greatest Role Model - That's kinda the job of a hero. That's why we all look up to them.

Many younger people look on Instagram and FaceBook for people to look up to. I'm here to tell you to stop just for today - you are awesome in your own right every single day! You are stronger than you know. You have so much determination to accomplish anything you want. You are *amazing*.

DO MORE OF WHAT MAKES YOU HAPPY

Think about this for a minute. When was the last time you asked yourself - what makes me happy?

I know we are all busy with things we have to do - jobs, kids, school, obligations ... the list goes on and on and on.

What makes you happy?

Do you do it enough?

If not, how can you fit it into your day or week so you are happier?

This does not have to be something big. It can be meeting with a friend for coffee every few weeks. Taking 20 minutes a day to walk your dog. Sitting down and reading a book for 30 minutes a day - despite what else you need to do!

I realized after my accident that I needed to do more things that make me happy. I am guilty of doing too much in a day - work, errands, working out, cooking- the whole mom thing. I realized in the last few years I didn't see my friends enough, and seeing my friends really makes me happy.

This year, I've seen more of my friends whether it's for coffee or to run together than I have in the last few years, and I am a much happier person. The simple acts of connecting with people I love fills up my emotional tank.

Look at your week this week. Try to add a few things to your calendar that make you happy!

BE THANKFUL FOR YOURSELF AND YOUR HEALTH

November is the month we see so many articles/posts about things to be thankful for in our lives. Our families, our friends, our pets – really the list is endless.

How often do you take the time to be thankful for yourself and your health?

Have you ever been thankful for yourself and your health?

I think Oprah started the gratitude journal idea many years ago and now it's everywhere. Start the day thinking about 3 things you are thankful for before you even get out of bed. It's not a terrible idea.

Our days are so busy and fast paced that taking a moment to think about just 3 things to be thankful for is a great way to start or end any/every day.

Today's message is about *you*. Stop the negative self-talk about what you are lacking/don't like about your physical/mental self, and *start* being thankful for yourself and your health every single day.

Many have it so much worse than you do right now. Unable to walk, get out of bed, have chronic pain, are sick - the list could take up the whole page, but you get the point.

Wherever you are right now - be thankful for all you are and celebrate yourself and your health. It could be worse, but right now it's not. You are awesome and amazing - that is worth being thankful for!

IT'S FINE

If you are a Grey's Anatomy fan, you know the words "I'm fine" or "It's fine" are said often. For many years it was Meredith and Christina (I totally miss her!) saying I'm fine, to each other. It never was fine. There was always some drama. Code words it's fine = not fine.

I'm not sure why, but in our society it seems we'd rather put up a front and say I'm fine even when we are not. We rarely say, "I'm not ok, I'm struggling, I need help." Why is that?

Certainly social media doesn't help. It seems we only see the amazing side of people's lives. We all go through ups and downs. I think most of us are willing and want to help others in need.

I certainly have been on the receiving end of that throughout the last year. I'm so thankful for all of my friends who pitched in and brought meals and texted me to see how I was doing. Those acts of kindness went a long way in making me feel better.

Next time you are struggling or need help - just ask! Your loved ones will be more than happy to help. I know I feel really great being able to help others and am guessing you do as well. No one is *fine* all the time. Take care of yourself and reach out to your friends. You'll feel better sooner than you think.

CONSISTENCY

I think anything you want to do well requires consistency. Think of any sport or hobby - you've got to practice on a regular basis if you want to see improvement.

I was just thinking back to when my kids took piano. I was amazed at their progression. They didn't always love to practice. But it really paid off as their skills improved dramatically with just a few hours spent at the piano each week.

The same goes for your health/fitness. I have known many people over the years that have gotten frustrated with their lack of results in a short time. They'd start a "diet" (I hate that word) and be upset if they didn't lose 5 lbs in the first week. They'd be convinced "dieting" doesn't work and why did nothing happen because they tried so hard ... for a few days! You cannot undo many days/months of less than optimal eating in just a week.

You know what? Dieting doesn't work. Making small changes really is the key to long term success. Consistency in moving your body, drinking water, getting your veggies in and getting enough rest. This is not glamorous or sexy, and definitely does not yield fast results. What this will do is result in lifelong success in your health. It's up to you to put in the work in on a daily/weekly basis.

Please value yourself and your health. Put your health on the top of your to-do list every single day. You are worth it!

NO

Happy crazy holiday season. Work, parties, decorating, cooking, friends, family – you know the drill. Busiest time of year for many of us.

That is why I want you to remember that "No" is a complete sentence. I don't want you to forget your own health this time of year. Now, more than ever, you need to keep yourself and your health at the top of your to do list every single day.

Sometimes we think we can do it all and then some, and be fine! If you are stretched too thin, just say no. No I can't, no thank you, no thanks or just plain No! These will all work, no further explanation is needed.

This time of year it's especially important to keep your health goals at the top of your list instead of waiting till January 1. No one really keeps New Year's resolutions anyway. I'd love for you to finish off the year exercising consistently and eating well.

It's not hard to do; you just need to say yes to your health every single day.

I WISH ...

Last night I was watching Terminator 2 with my kids. It originally came out in 1991. I was 24 years old. I remember watching it and thinking OMG, I wish I had Linda Hamilton's arms. I wish I could do a pull-up!

We all see things that we wish we could do, right?

How often do we actually take steps to follow through and make that wish a reality?

I was a runner for many years. I didn't really think about strength training until my late 40's. I had crazy arm envy but did nothing about it. It wasn't until I was 46 - yup 22 years later that I actually started working on pull-ups. I'm reading that last line looking at how ridiculous that looks. I waited 22 years to work on something I really wanted to do. That's just stupid.

If you want something, don't wish for it! Start working towards it now! Today and tomorrow, and don't stop until you reach your goal.

And yes, I can do pull ups now because I work on them on a regular basis. It's pretty awesome, I must admit. But it's ridiculous to wait *so long* to do something that you really want. I do not have Linda Hamilton arms, but I can bust out some amazing pull ups!

MAKING HEALTHY CHOICES IS NOT HARD

We are doing the Whole 30 in my house for the month of January. One of my daughter's role models is Emily Boyd (@eboydsfood on Instagram) who just recently finished the Whole 30 in December. Emily is a former keeper for the Cal Berkeley women's soccer team. Emily is a stud! She posts her killer workouts, as well as lots of amazing meals. This inspired my daughter to want to try the Whole 30.

Emily has been posting pics of her meals for months now on IG. In December she committed to the Whole 30 and loved how this plan made her feel. This is a gal who already was an incredibly healthy eater and in amazing shape! All her meals looked awesome - they are loaded with veggies, eggs, meats and avocados! So colorful they always make me smile.

Short version - no added sugar (or sugar of any kind- honey, stevia, etc.), no gluten, dairy, grains, booze or processed foods. What can you eat? Meats, healthy fats (avocados, nuts) all veggies and fruits. Coffee is ok (thank goodness or else it'd be a hard pass from me). Eat one ingredient foods and see great things happen in 30 days.

I cannot tell you how much I love what the gal who created the Whole 30 says about this program: "Don't you dare tell me this is hard. Beating cancer is hard. Birthing a baby is hard. Losing a parent is hard. You've done harder things than this and you have no excuse not to complete this program as written. It's only 30 days, and it's for the most important health cause on earth: the only physical body you will ever have in this lifetime."

Here's a gal who says exactly how I feel about taking care of yourself. I've heard every excuse out there as to why someone can't take care of themselves. It really isn't hard. And it is a choice - one you make every day, every time you eat, every time you move your body.

Are there roadblocks? You bet! Every single time you go into a coffee shop, you are given many yummy drinks to choose from. We just finished the holidays where special treats and big meals are part of that time of year. Treats at work overflow - it's always someone's birthday right?

Here's the deal - we do only have one body to go through life with. Take care of yourself and your health. You will feel better day in and day out, year in and year out if you move your body and eat well.

YOUR COMFORT ZONE

Last week I went to my favorite yoga teacher's 90 minute class. Before taking yoga at his studio, I never "got" yoga. I tried it a few times at different gyms. I just didn't get when I'd hear people say that it was the best part of their day. Really?

Then a friend brought me to East Wind Yoga. My whole view of yoga changed. Scott the owner is an exceptional teacher. I am super picky when it comes to taking classes - yoga or otherwise. Because I've been a teacher for so long, I only will take from really good teachers.

Scott is a stickler for excellent form. He challenges students every single time they walk through his door. In his 90 minute class last Thursday I was so out of my comfort zone both mentally and physically. It was a battle to hold the poses he was asking us to do. The strength work was also super hard. Tiny movements that left me in a puddle of my own sweat. The mind controls the body and it was a challenging night for me.

I left feeling energized! I fought hard and made it through. I knew I needed to do that once a week. I need to get out of my own comfort zone and be challenged. What doesn't challenge you doesn't change you - right??

This week, my challenge for you is to get out of your comfort zone. Try something new. Or put more effort into your workout. Try to push yourself mentally and physically to see how you feel. After you do, email me to let me know how it went!

It's way easier to stay in your comfort zone but I promise you it will be worth it if you step out of it!

HARD WORK

I teach one class a week. It's a functional class with lots of core work, squats, balance and strength. This class is attended mostly by seniors. I think the youngest in this class is 55 and goes up to the 70's.

We all lose muscle mass as we age. This is just a fact of life. We also lose our balance. This is why so many older people fall down and break their hips and other bones.

I always chuckle when I see the advice that tells you to stand on one foot when you brush your teeth! Come on - really? Disaster waiting to happen right there. However, we all need to work on balance and strength - every week if possible.

I am a hard teacher. If you take time out of your day to come workout with me, I want it to be worth it! I want you to leave feeling accomplished and proud of yourself. This also goes for my current class. I do not take it easy on them because I want them to reap the benefits of strength training!

One member told me that since taking my class her knees no longer hurt when she bent down to get clothes out of the dryer. Another said for the first time on her annual deep sea fishing trip, she could reel the fish in without any help! That to me is music to my ears.

Just this last Friday, a student said to me, "You were really hard on us today. I didn't like it, but know in a few days I will be thankful that you did."

Are you working hard enough? I'm just asking because I see *so many* people at the gym barely working. Our bodies were meant to work hard. I'm not saying every day but at least a few days a week- go harder than you want to. Lift heavier weights, take a class that is challenging (maybe yoga?), try to walk/run outside. Get out of head and try, just try to do more.

ATTITUDE

Last weekend my husband and I were talking about our plans for the day. I said I was going out for a run. He said that he wished he could run outside with me. Because of many knee surgeries, he can't do this.

The exception is when on vacation - we run hills together. This is a man who doesn't run on a regular basis. I've been a runner for 40 years. He always beats me on hill repeats. Smiling, laughing at me and sometimes running backwards just to prove that he's still got it! Those are some fun times.

I told him I was heading out and always think how thankful I am to run. Even if I'm only going out for a few miles, it's awesome to be able to run. A year ago, I was still recovering from my accident and couldn't run yet. I try to remember how lucky I am and enjoy every run!

Then I left the house. It's cold. Even though I grew up in Ohio, I am a wimp. I wear mittens at 50 degrees. My seat heater is on much of the year in my car. I know it's a lot colder in many parts of the country.

It didn't warm up. There was nothing good about this run. My face was cold, my nose was running, it was really damn cold.

I may have said some swear words in regards to how cold it was and how I felt. More than a few.

Then it hit me like a ton of bricks. I sounded like a petulant little 5 year old brat! Oh it's cold! Oh my face is cold! Boo-fricken-hoo!

Didn't I just tell my husband that I was thankful to be running? Immediate change of attitude- STAT!

I'm thankful to be running. My body is healthy and strong. I CAN run. If things had been different, I may never have been able to run again. The last mile was spent in gratitude. Not being a whiny brat. Needless to say, it was a great run.

So many things can be changed with a positive or grateful attitude. Try it! Let me know the results as I always like to hear from you!

HARD TRUTH

Just today I was at my gym overheard this conversation that went something like this:

"What are you doing in here on a Sunday?"

The reply: "It's Superbowl and we made chicken wings and cheese sticks. I have to burn it all off now."

I'm cringing inside as I'm hearing this. Now before you get mad at me for telling you the truth, I'm not against eating chicken wings or cheese sticks. In fact, in college I worked at a bar that made amazing wings. Every shift I worked, I would dip wings in blue cheese dressing and hot sauce (along with curly fries as well)! Heaven in my mouth.

I was cringing because the myth people still believe is ... if I workout, I can eat whatever I want. Not true.

Here's what people underestimate - the amount of calories burned. The workout is always a great idea don't get me wrong. It's just that many use it as a reason to eat far more than what they burned in the gym.

In fact, I was at my heaviest in college when I was running marathons. Yes, you read that correctly. In addition to running loads of miles a week, I was eating dorm food, subs, pizza and my beloved chicken wings and Egg McMuffins. I did eat salad ... with cheese and blue cheese dressing and croutons.

You can't out-exercise a fork. I am always going to tell you the truth about health and fitness. I don't want you to not indulge. I want you to enjoy and celebrate fun times. I also don't want you to wake up with a food hangover - those are the worst and yes, I've had many of them myself!

I am here to lead you down the path of health. I see so many people taking their health for granted and treating their bodies like a garbage can - I want more for you!

MOTIVATION

I just received an email asking how to get motivated to go to the gym. This is something I've been asked many times over the years.

I believe it's easier to stay motivated for your workouts if you *love* what you do.

If you just go to the gym to get it in and get no joy out of it, then it's easy to skip or find a reason not to go.

It's also important to have a *why*. A big picture *why*. I tell my clients to write it on a sticky note and post it everywhere - car, desk, bathroom to remind yourself why you are going to the gym even when you don't want to.

If hitting the gym and doing the cardio equipment/weights isn't your thing, find an activity you love that gets you moving. There's no shortage of classes offered - cross fit, zumba, boot camp, yoga - the list is endless. I also find that people stay consistent if they have a friend/group of people to hold them accountable.

There are times when I need motivation as well believe it or not! This last year was rough and two things really helped. Running with my girlfriends is the first. It was such fun to get out there and get moving, talk and laugh and get coffee afterwards.

The second thing that really helped me was FitRadio. I found this app last spring. It has a coaching feature where a coach tells me what to do and motivates me along the way. This literally saved my running. I had to start and stop working out so much last year, I just couldn't get motivated to go out and run a few miles. FitRadio made it *fun* and challenging and there are different workouts each week. The coaching is also available for indoor cardio - bike, elliptical, treadmill etc.

I recently went ice-skating with a girlfriend. We both grew up skating and I've always loved it. It was so much fun and great to do something I don't normally do. We now have a 2X a month date to keep it up. Was I awesome? Nope - but it came back slowly and I was so happy I got back on the ice after too many years off it.

It's up to you to find what you love doing and keep going. We only have one body to go through life with - why not take the best care of it that you can. That means regular movement every single day. It's doesn't have to be boring or a burden. Grab a friend and go for a walk- that's moving! Just don't stop - ever.

HOW TO EAT

I just recently had a friend message me about eating. She is trying to lose weight and is so confused. There is so much conflicting information out there. She is overwhelmed.

Eat for your body shape, eat for your blood type, eat for your age, eat for heart health, eat what the government says to eat (please don't do that one)! The list is literally endless.

I listen to lots of health gurus thru podcasts and have for years. These are people from all different arenas - Neurologists, Plant Based Experts, Wellness Experts to name a few. There may be some differences, but they all have a few rules they all swear by as far as eating for weight loss:

1. Eat a lot of veggies. Every single person who I've ever listened to has this on their list. Most recommend 2-6 servings of veggies per day and 2-3 servings of in season fruit. We tend to hear eat your fruits and veggies. All the gurus say, eat more veggies than fruit and eat tons of vegetables.

2. Avoid processed foods. So much of what comes out of a package contains chemicals that are not great for our bodies. It's a fact of life that sometimes we all eat packaged food - just read your

labels carefully. Stick with unprocessed real foods as much as possible.

3. Eat healthy fats. The 80's threw our country for a loop with the whole "fat is bad" theme. The sugar free theme created so many health problems we are still dealing with today. Taking out the fat but adding a ton of sugar = so much heart disease, and let's not forget the obesity epidemic. Real fat is vital to our bodies - our brains need fat as it is made up of 60% fat. Fatty fish, avocado, nuts and seeds are great for our bodies, brains, as well as hair skin and nails.

4. Limit sugar. Sorry to be the bearer of this news if this is new to you. Sugar is not awesome for our bodies. Pick and choose your sugar wisely. I'm not going to list the all the reasons it's not great for us, just eat mostly real food, and sugar in moderation.

5. Drink water. Although not food related - we all need water every single day. Our bodies are made up of about 70% water - start drinking to support all your organs and body's needs. Start drinking water when you get up and always have your glass or water bottle by your side! Don't leave home without your water bottle.

Here's a quick tip - every meal should have protein (meat, fish, beans, quinoa, tofu, etc), healthy fats, healthy carbs (sweet potato, potato, rice, fruit, veg) - that is it.

It shouldn't be hard to know what to eat to lose weight. But, with the overabundance of information out there, I understand how it can be confusing!

If you need more information than this, check out my book *The Rules for Weight Loss* where I go more in depth on this topic. Check it out on my website – theperfectbalance.guru.

INSANITY

Do you know the definition of insanity?

It is doing the same thing over and over and over and expecting different results.

Have you ever been there?

I've seen it a lot. People who complain about their health (more often complain about themselves), try to do the same thing they always do, and never get the results they are looking for.

If there is some aspect of your life or your health that you don't like, change it. I realize this is so much easier said than done. However, you are the only one in charge of yourself and your health. The *only* one.

I had a client years ago who told me many times how unhappy she was with her weight - on a weekly basis. I finally asked her what she was doing about it. She told me "nothing" was working. But when pressed, she admitted she hadn't changed anything at all. She told me her husband finally said to her, "If you're not happy, do something about it or stop complaining!" (In a loving way of course!)

It was an eye opening moment for her. For me as well. Over the years, most of my clients have been somewhat unhappy with their physical appearance. Doing the work and making a commitment to themselves to change was the hard part; complaining was the easy part.

Here's my challenge to you this week. Think about what you complain about the most. Either do something about it or stop complaining about it. That's it.

If you need help figuring out how to change, just shoot me an email - I am here to help! We all (myself included) have things we complain about and could improve!

What if you actually took steps to improve the one thing that really bugs you? You may feel like a million bucks!

BE HAPPY NOW

Be happy now. Sounds simple right? But ... how many times have you said to yourself, "I'll be happy when (fill in the blank)." A few examples: when I lose weight, when I start exercising, when I start eating better, this weekend, after I finish all my work, after I finish delivering Girl Scout cookies. The list is endless.

Gratitude is a game changer. It's for everyone. Gratitude turns perspective around faster than anything else.

As a trainer for a long time, I cringe when I hear clients say, "I will be happy when I lose weight. Why not choose happy now?"

If you don't like the way you feel in your own skin, do something about it. But choose happy every single day. Your life will be better because of it. Depression and despair will just make you (and everyone around you) miserable.

Bear with me as I play devil's advocate for a moment.

- Can you walk?
- Are you reasonable healthy?
- Do you have people in your life who you love and love you back?

- Can you move your body without pain?
- Can you bite into an apple?

Ok, the last one was just for me to crack myself up because I cannot bite into any food yet – not until I get my permanent teeth. But you get the picture. Be happy today. Don't let your weight, your expectations of yourself, or your daily grind get you down. Your day will be better when you choose happiness.

SET YOURSELF UP FOR SUCCESS

I want to talk about being successful in the health and fitness game.

I just had coffee with a few girlfriends the other day. One of them was so hard on herself because she didn't get up early on a Saturday to take a class. This friend is not a morning person. She doesn't like getting up early to workout, let alone on a Saturday. She's setting herself up for failure.

I suggested she go out for a run or run walk later in the day. She did and lo and behold she felt amazing! Knowing what works for you can make all the difference in the world in your health and fitness.

I see this far too often. People setting themselves up for failure. Just recently another friend who is trying to lose weight commented she had just downed a couple boxes of Girl Scout cookies in a few days. She felt awful.

Um, ok I get that you want to support the Girl Scouts but if you're trying to lose weight and cannot control yourself (around

Thin Mints - who can?), don't bring them into your house! You can buy the cookies and send them to the military overseas - a great option if you cannot be trusted with an open box of cookies!

The same goes for exercise. If you are not a morning person, don't think you're going to get out of bed and workout before your day starts. Hitting the alarm, sleeping until you have to get up and beating yourself up for not working out is just an awful way to go through any day.

Know when the best time to work out is for you and do it then. Know what your trigger foods are and don't keep them around if you can't stop eating them. We are all human, not robots.

Set yourself up for success by knowing what works for you and what doesn't. Your whole day will be so much better and you will be happier with yourself and your health by doing so.

GIVE YOURSELF THE CREDIT YOU DESERVE

Are you hard on yourself?

Are you laughing right now because *of course* you are hard on yourself?

We are all our own worst critics by far. This can be a great thing as well as not so great.

If you are setting goals for yourself and you fall short, it's okay to be upset with yourself and make plans to reach them another way.

However, if you are constantly beating yourself up, that serves no purpose. You have to give yourself credit where credit is due.

For example, I just went to the track with my daughter to run some intervals. This was a regular thing for me in my 30's and 40's. I haven't done this in over 2 years. Intervals are hard work.

The first thing my mind went to is what awful shape I'm in. I have to reel myself in and know that first of all I'm doing my best.

Secondly, it's hard work and going to take a long time to build back my stamina. Last of all, I should give myself some credit for just showing up and doing it.

Instead of beating yourself up for not achieving x, y or z, give yourself a pat on the back for what you do each and every day. We are all doing some good things every day. Think about the good, and try to improve the not so good.

I GET TO WORK OUT TODAY!

Earlier this week, I had an unexpected procedure on my mouth. My periodontist told me that I couldn't work out for 5 days. He knows me well after working with me for 16 months now. He knows I need an exact number of days, as I will be back at it as soon as I can!

I've had more time off in the last year from exercising than I have since I started running when I was 11! I've had to take anywhere from a week off to 3 weeks off from exercise after each of my surgeries. This to me, is the worst side effect of the accident.

To me, exercise is a part of my daily life. I feel better when I exercise. It helps me sort out the craziness in my life. My whole day goes better when I exercise. I am a better mom and wife when I exercise. I've never found it hard to fit it in. I make it a priority because of how it makes me feel.

Today when I was finally able to work out, I was so thankful. Exercise makes me happy. My body just likes to move. I know many look at exercise as a chore and don't/can't find time to fit it into their day.

Some people look at exercise and think, uggghhh I have to work out today. If they don't work out, they feel guilty. Too much time off from exercise and it's easy to find other things to do in your day.

How do you feel right now in your body?

You get to work out every single day if you want to! Walking counts, Zumba counts, yoga counts, any kind of movement counts. Our bodies were meant to move so get out there today and get moving!

If you struggle getting motivated, here's a thought for you. Don't look at exercise like a chore. Look at it like a vital and necessary part of your day. It should be non-negotiable to take care of your health every single day. You will feel better in your body if you move it- so get moving!

HAPPY BIRTHDAY

It's my 51st birthday in 2 days. This year I decided to get myself a present in February. I got myself a trainer!

Why, you ask would I hire a trainer when I myself am a trainer?

I have goals for myself this year and knew I needed help. I realized what I wanted to accomplish was outside my area of expertise. It's been great and fun in a painful way. I lost a lot of muscle last year. I wanted help in building back the muscle.

It's been awesome not to have to think about what I need to do for a workout. To be told and pushed and pushed is just what I needed.

I am guilty of staying in my comfort zone when I lifted in the past. I'd make a workout around what I liked. I would push myself a little but not enough to get the results I am looking for.

Are you satisfied with where you are physically right now?

If the answer is no, go out and get someone who can help you get there. It is always helpful to have someone hold you accountable and take you to the next level.

If it's the food you need help with, start keeping a food log. Myfitnesspal is a great way to track what you eat. Get a friend who is also logging and hold each other accountable. Success comes from accountability.

SETBACKS

We will all at one time or another face a setback. It could be big or small. They stink. No doubt about it.

What can you do?

Don't be too hard on yourself and please don't give up.

Just do what you can each day and try to stay consistent.

It's better to aim for progress, not perfection. Your health is worth your time and effort every day.

I have had loads of setbacks this past year. More than in my whole life combined. It was frustrating and annoying and awful. But I got through by just doing what I could every day. Some days were literally spent on the couch. Some days I could walk my dog around the block.

There used to be this great guy at the gym where I used to work. He would scream at the top of his lungs - "Better than Yesterday!" every single day. This guy had been in a serious car accident, almost died, had loads of metal in his body and was in pain a lot. But, he did what he could, stayed positive and inspired all of us who were with him.

Don't let a setback get you off track permanently. One step at a time, one day at a time.

There's no such thing as a good excuse for not taking care of yourself.

SERIOUSLY

I've been dealing with an infection in my mouth for the last 6 weeks. It's not been painful, just really annoying as I thought all the hard stuff was over with.

Today my awesome periodontist got to the bottom of it. There was a lot of cutting into my gums, about an hours' worth, as well as more bone grafting. He told let me know I need to get a root canal ASAP so the infection doesn't come back.

I actually went into today with a positive attitude determined not to let whatever came up get me down. It's amazing how far this took me. My doctor and his nurse commented that I was beyond a doubt their most positive patient in the practice.

My reply was, it's better than being dead. Which was my mantra in 2017. Still holds true today. No matter what else I have to go through I am still here.

After the procedure, I had to go to the store. I couldn't have my cat yelling at me tomorrow for running out of food. Those of you that have cats totally get this. There was also some meds to pick up.

At that point, the Novocain was just wearing off and I was in a good amount of pain. I had downed some ibuprofen but it had not kicked in yet.

As I am checking out, I heard this woman talking rather harshly to the self-checkout attendant. It went something like this. "I *cannot* believe this store doesn't carry *cold* Diet Dr. Pepper. It's really what I want right now and I can't have it."

SERIOUSLY!

It took every ounce of will power to hold my tongue. After that, I just felt sorry for her. This is what she's complaining about.

Be positive, look at the bright side of things and be thankful for everything you have - not what you don't have!

BAD DAYS

Today started off as a bad day. I was grumpy last night, had a bad night's sleep and woke up grumpy today.

I knew why. I had a dermatologist appointment. I've had 2 skin cancer moles dug out of me in last 6 months.

This is because my goal in the 80's was to be as tan as possible. Every vacation in North Carolina was filled with hours of laying out and body surfing. As was every spring break trip to Florida. There was no such thing as sunscreen, just tanning lotion and oil.

In college, we used to lie out on top of the parking garages and houses so we could get closer to the sun. If you're laughing while reading this – it's true. If you did this also, I'm sure you are laughing as well.

The smell of Hawaiian Tropic or Ban de Soleil still makes me smile and think of vacation. I rarely burned as my mom is Italian. Instead, I got really, really tan.

Now, I'm paying the price for all those hours of basking in the sun. I woke up today thinking, I just can't take it. I cannot take any more digging into my body. I've had *enough* digging to last a lifetime.

I went for a warm up run - or should I say sprint before my workout. I ran as fast as I could to try to run the bad feelings out. Then I lifted a lot of weight and did a lot of pull ups. This helped.

Turns out, I did have an abnormal mole. My dermatologist dug a bit for a biopsy. I have no expectations anymore. They crush me. I should know by Friday whether it needs to be really dug out or I am good. Either way, it's better than dead as was my motto last year.

The rest of the day was great. I had a meeting with some fabulous women who I am doing a speaking event with this month. Then had lunch with a girlfriend.

The best part of my day was seeing my periodontist outside of his office. His wife had just had a baby and he was out getting food. I remember him telling me when they found out that they were pregnant. Today I got to hear the birth story. I'm heading over in a bit to bring him cookies and green smoothies!

Getting out of my own head and being with others really does help when you're feeling down. So does exercise.

Next time you're having a bad day, go get your sweat on! Then call a friend or two and get out of your house and into the fresh air. It will pass.

P.S.- The mole was NOT cancer. I was surprised!

DEFINITION OF HARD

In case you didn't know I'm a *huge* running geek. I've been a runner for 40 years now. When my friends post pics on Facebook of their kids running track, I always want to know what events they ran and their times. Yes, I still want to know the details!

The Boston Marathon was a few weeks ago. I always look forward to reading about the athletes running as well as special interest stories.

In that week's Sacramento Bee and New York Times, there was an article on Tim Don. He's the world record holder in the Ironman. That race is a 2.1 mile ocean swim, 112 mile bike ride and finishes with a 26.2 mile run. Ouch!

He was hit by a car and got what is known as a hangman's fracture. A broken C-2 vertebrae. He could have had surgery to fix it. This would have been easy and comfortable. But it would limit his neck's range of motion thereby ending his athletic career.

He chose instead to have the halo. This is an excruciating experience, but the best option for a full recovery. Tim chose this method because he wanted to continue competing. Titanium pins were screwed into his skull, 2 in the front and 2 in the back, and attach them to metal bars which attaches to a bust that you wear for 3 months that you can't take off. To say it's painful is putting it mildly.

His goal was to run the Boston Marathon in under 2:50. This was the time of the marathon he ran in his last Ironman competition. The weather was awful for the race. Cold icy rain and headwinds that greeted all the runners on the hills of Boston. His time was 2:49.

Now let's talk about what your goals are and if you think they are hard ...

I'm certain you can do anything you put your mind to. You just have to decide your goal is worth fighting for.

I see people fail at their goals all the time. The goal isn't too hard. It's what it takes to reach it that is looked at as too hard. What's worse - sacrificing to reach your goal or not reaching it at all?

WHAT CAN HAPPEN IN A YEAR

Do you ever look back and think wow – a lot has happened in the last year?

A year ago, I had a major mouth surgery. After every surgery, I had to take time off from working out. Following each surgery, when my body was up for it, I'd get back into exercise. It was so good for not only my physical but my mental state as well.

I have a pull up bar in my back yard. I have always wanted to do pull ups. I put a picture of a woman doing a pull up on my vision board when I was 37! It wasn't until 10 years after that, that I actually started working on pull ups and was able to do one.

After my accident, my sports guru said to lay off the pull ups as I was straining my neck. Mind you, I wasn't doing many of them but clearly was leading up with my chin and messing myself up. I really didn't mind stopping, I just wanted what was best for my body.

Then I was having a conversation with my son's trainer (now my trainer) and he said – there's nothing wrong with sets of 1 when it comes to pull ups. This was mind blowing. It made so much sense in my case. I can do one. I started adding them back into my workouts literally one at a time.

In the last few months, I've worked up to sets of 2, then 3. Last weekend, my trainer had me do 25 total in a workout. I thought he was crazy. Spread out over an hour workout was actually doable.

This week, he told me I was going to do 40. Again– really? Ok – he knows what people are capable of ... That 40 turned into 51. Over the course of 90 minutes. There were many sets of one.

When I told my husband, he reminded me that a year ago, I wasn't even doing one pull up. It was an eye opening moment.

We can all grow in a year. It just depends on putting the work in on a daily/weekly basis.

What do you want to do in the next year?

You are stronger than you know.

LIFE CHOICES

Last week I had to take my car in to get new tires. The guy behind the counter had an open container of berries and cantaloupe on the counter.

We started talking and I said - sorry to interrupt your snack. He laughed and said - it's fine, part of the new diet I am on.

Of course I asked about his new diet!

He replied, "Clearly I need it," as he put his hands on his sizable belly. "It's actually pretty good. I eat lots of fruit and veggies and drink a ton of water." He told me that it's surprising how his taste buds have changed.

He used to eat a lot of pizza and burgers. He told me that he did this all to himself and now he is paying the price.

Then he said, he just had had a burger this week. Funny thing, it didn't taste as good as he remembered. He was really surprised by this as he used to love burgers. Also taking him by surprise is how good fruit tastes.

This isn't the first time I've heard this. Often times, the hardest part (of taking on a new eating plan) is breaking up with foods that don't serve you well. A once in a while burger/junk food/etc. is fine. The guy helping me had over 50+ pounds to lose.

Fast food/chips/cookies/any processed food are made to entice us to keep eating and eating and eating. They make it that way on purpose! Can't have just one - Lay's slogan - but it's true. Who can have just one chip?

If you have weight to lose, try breaking up with whatever food you know is not awesome for your health. It won't be easy, and the first few days, you may feel lousy. But then, you'll feel great.

Food is here to mostly nourish our bodies. Sometimes for fun, but mostly for fuel. Think about how you feel on a daily basis. Try to eat more foods that will give you energy then make you crash.

SUCK IT UP, BUTTERCUP

If you've ever been in my class or a client of mine, you are cracking up right now. This is an expression I use a lot. Especially if I think you need a good kick in the behind.

Today, I had to say this to myself. It's been a rough week. I had the last procedure done on my mouth (hopefully). I'm a year and 5 months into my recovery and really hoping this is it. Whenever I get work done on my mouth, it sidelines me for days.

I literally can't do much except nap, read, and rest. Maybe a short dog walk. I have no desire or energy to workout. If you don't know me personally, I have to tell you this is the exact opposite of my normal self. I typically have a hard time taking a day off from exercise. My body (and mind) just love to move.

This morning I asked my husband what the weather was like. He had just come from getting the paper outside. He looked at me and said, it's a great day for a run. Meaning - Suck it UP Buttercup and get yourself out there and move. He didn't verbally say this, but after being married for 22 years, his eyes said it all. I replied that it's a nice day for someone else to run ... I had no desire to run.

But I knew this was one of those times. Suck it up and get moving. I did. I told my family I was going out to run a mile. It was nice to be moving again. Then I lifted a bit in my backyard. Nothing crazy, but a little more movement.

I felt SO good the rest of the day. I was super productive. I have a bunch of projects going on right now and made a big dent in my to-do list – even though it's a Sunday. I had enough rest this week – it's time to get stuff done.

Moral of the story – sometimes you need a good kick in the behind from someone else or yourself to get going. Once you get going, you will be happy you did. Every single time.

THERE IS NO "THERE"

I have heard many times over the years, "when I lose weight then I will... (fill in the blank)." Usually something along these lines - buy some new clothes, feel better about myself, go paddleboarding (or any water activity), wear shorts, take an active vacation ... you get the picture.

So often people look at weight loss (and for that matter a healthy life) with an end point. Once I lose the weight, I can go off my diet. Once I lose my weight, I can stop with all the exercise. Once I reach my health goal, I can stop working so hard.

I am here to tell you there is no stopping. Health and wellness is a lifelong journey. There is no end while you are above ground.

I've seen it too often over the years. Clients, close friends, even family members lose weight and/or make great changes to their health. They always feel amazing! Every single time.

Then slowly, old habits creep back into their daily lives. The weight starts creeping up little by little. Before they know it, they are back where they started or even worse off than when they started.

It's a job to take care of your health. The most important one you will ever have. Keep putting yourself at the top of your to do list every single day. You are worth it. You will feel better – I promise.

Now, I want you to promise me that you will never give up on your health journey. Even when you think you are at your "goal." Keep on plugging along and making those good choices. It will always be worth it. Every single time.

THERE ARE NO SHORTCUTS

I was at my gym this week talking to one of my clients. He asked me about what's going on with my teeth. I told him what the latest was as well as that I'm about 6 weeks away from getting my real teeth.

A guy who I do not know asked me if I was the one having work done on my teeth. I said yes and told him I have implants and currently in a bridge. He told me I should go to Mexico. Not only is it cheaper, but it's so much faster than what you can get done here.

I tried nicely to explain that I have unusual circumstances and it's been a long journey. He would not stop. I could really save a lot of money and time if I'd go to Mexico. In fact, he got his implants in one day. I had enough, so I just smiled and wished him luck and walked away.

In my head, I was thinking - are you kidding me? There are no shortcuts with your teeth. For that matter with your health, with your diet, with your exercise plan. None of those things can be achieved by any short cuts.

I texted my periodontist about this guy and his response was this ..."I love when they go. They always end up being taken out by me within a year. It's more expensive to take out implants and rebuild the damage than placing them right the first time." We had a good laugh over this.

I hope you know by now that there are no quick fixes, no short cuts. Anything worth having takes time. But it's so worth your time to do it right! Take the time for yourself and your health every single day.

Your health is your wealth!

REASONS OR RESULTS

I was just listening to a podcast the other day. One line really resonated with me. It had to do with reaching your goals. The person being interviewed said, "People either have reasons why they don't reach their goals or they have results."

Wow!

That made a lot of sense. Some people put their nose to the grindstone and work. They don't stop working until they are done. Others make excuses as to why they can't work/finish/reach their goal.

This applies to all areas of life, including health and fitness.

Which one are you?

We all have the power to change. If you want something bad enough, you will do what is necessary to get there. Be awesome. Make big changes. Feel amazing. You are the only one in control of your health destiny.

IT'S NOT A CHORE

Today I was at the bank taking care of some business. The banker helping me was great. I was there for a while and we got to talking about a few things.

He asked what I drank as I had a Starbucks cup. I told him I'm boring and get the same thing - Grande Americano with some cold soy milk.

I asked him what he drank from Starbucks as it's literally next door to the bank. He said he didn't get anything from there as he drinks his coffee at home. We got to talking about the specialty drinks. I said I just can't afford that much sugar/calories in a drink. I said I'm "old" (older than him) and I'd rather eat my calories than drink them.

He told me I'm not old. But looked at my account that had my birthdate. He said I was the same age as his dad - 50. I asked if his dad did anything special for his big 5-0 and he replied no. He asked me how I celebrated mine. I told him I got my best adult friends together to play kickball. We then brought the party back to my house for dinner.

He looked sad and said his dad doesn't make good choices. He looks at taking care of himself as a chore. Seeing his dad not taking care of his health inspired him to start making different choices. He showed me his Fitbit and told me what his daily goal is for steps.

The point is, good health is a choice we all make every single day, not a chore! So many people look at taking care of themselves as an insurmountable chore. Really?

We all have things to take care of: kids, house, job, pets, husbands (lol). All kidding aside, putting yourself at the top of the list should mandatory. How on earth can you take care of anyone else if you don't take care of yourself?

How do you feel right now?

If you don't feel awesome, make a few better choices today. And then a few more tomorrow. Strive for progress, not perfection.

AGE IS JUST A NUMBER

My cousin just forwarded me a video clip on Facebook that was incredible.

It was about Ida Keeling. She's a 102 year old amazing woman. She started running at 67 after her daughter signed her up for a race. Now, she's breaking records pretty much every time she runs. She was the only woman in 2016 to run 100 meters at the age of 100.

She lost 2 kids around the same time and fell into a deep depression. She says exercise is one of the best medications. One of her best quotes is "Don't sit around and do nothing." Her secret to living a long life is "running, a big breakfast and a sip of cognac."

So many times in life we limit ourselves. We think we can't do something. This lady started running at 67. What can't you do?

Get out of your comfort zone, try something new, move your body and know that exercise really is the best medication!

MORE INFO

Go to theperfectbalance.guru to join my "Sexy in 60 Days" program and get a free gift! You can also sign up for more weekly inspirations like these by subscribing to my weekly newsletter, "The Perfect Balance Bulletin."